# MICROBIOME
# COOKBOOK

## MAIN COURSE - Breakfast, Lunch, Dinner and Dessert Recipes to restore your gut health

# TABLE OF CONTENTS

purposes solely, and is universal as so. The presentation of the information is without contract or any type of guarantee assurance.

The trademarks that are used are without any consent, and the publication of the trademark is without permission or backing by the trademark owner. All trademarks and brands within this book are for clarifying purposes only and are the owned by the owners themselves, not affiliated with this document.


Introduction

Microbiome recipes for personal enjoyment but also for family enjoyment. You will love them for sure for how easy it is to prepare them.

# BREAKFAST

## ARUGULA & PEAR SMOOTHIE BOWL

Serves:        *2*
Prep Time:   *10*   Minutes

Cook Time:   *10*   Minutes

Total Time:   *20*   Minutes

### INGREDIENTS

- 1 cup arugula
- 1 kale leaf
- 2 cups romaine lettuce
- ¼ cup coconut water
- 1 tablespoon almond butter
- 1 pear
- 1 tablespoon chia seeds
- 1 tablespoon lemon juice

### DIRECTIONS

1. In a blender add all ingredients and blend until smooth

2. Blend for 2-3 minutes
3. When ready pour mixture into 2 bowls
4. Garnish with favorite topping and serve

Serves:      **4**
Prep Time:   **5**   Minutes

Cook Time:   **5**   Minutes

Total Time:  **10**  Minutes

## INGREDIENTS

- ¼ banana
- ¼ cup raspberries
- 1 cup coconut milk
- ¼ avocado
- ¼ cup Greek yogurt
- 1 tsp ginger
- ¼ cup ice

## DIRECTIONS

1. In a blender place all ingredients and blend until smooth
2. Pour smoothie in a glass and serve

# OVERNIGHT OATS WITH CHIA SEEDS

Serves:        **1**
Prep Time:     **5**   Minutes
Cook Time:     **15**  Minutes
Total Time:    **20**  Minutes

## INGREDIENTS

- ¼ cup chia seeds
- ¼ cup oats
- ¼ cup coconut milk
- 4 oz. Greek yogurt
- ¼ tsp cinnamon
- 1 tablespoon sweetened coconut

## DIRECTIONS

1. In a bowl add coconut milk, yogurt, cinnamon, oats, chia seeds and cover overnight
2. In a frying pan fry coconut for 3-4 minutes
3. Add fried coconut to oats and serve

# BANANA OVERNIGHT OATS WITH CHIA

Serves:          **1**

Prep Time:    **5**    Minutes

Cook Time:    **5**    Minutes

Total Time:   **10**   Minutes

## INGREDIENTS

- 1 banana
- 1 cup almond milk
- ¼ cup Greek yogurt
- 1 cup oats
- 1 tablespoon chia seeds
- 1 tablespoon almond butter

## DIRECTIONS

1. In a bowl add almond milk, Greek yogurt, oats, banana, chia seeds and almond butter
2. Refrigerate overnight
3. Serve in the morning

# SIMPLE OMELET

Serves:        **1**

Prep Time:    **5**   Minutes

Cook Time:   **10**   Minutes

Total Time:   **15**   Minutes

## INGREDIENTS

- 2 eggs
- salt
- 2 tablespoons butter
- ¼ cup cheddar cheese
- 1 tablespoon chives

## DIRECTIONS

1. In a bowl beat eggs with salt
2. Add remaining ingredients and mix well
3. In a skillet met butter and pour mixture
4. Cook for 1-2 minutes per side
5. When ready remove and serve

# CHEESESTEAK OMELET

Serves: **2**

Prep Time: **10** Minutes

Cook Time: **20** Minutes

Total Time: **30** Minutes

## INGREDIENTS

- 2 tablespoons olive oil
- 1 onion
- 2 bell peppers
- 6 oz. mushrooms
- ¼ sirloin steak
- 4 eggs
- 2 tablespoons milk
- 1 cup provolone

## DIRECTIONS

1. In a skillet heat olive oil and sauté peppers, mushrooms and onion

2. Add steak and cook for 2-3 minute per side
3. Add the rest of the ingredients and cook until steak has formed a crust
4. When ready remove from heat and serve

# POTATO OMELET

Serves: **2**

Prep Time: **10** Minutes

Cook Time: **10** Minutes

Total Time: **20** Minutes

## INGREDIENTS

- 6 eggs
- 2 cups potato chips
- ¼ cup parsley
- ¼ tsp salt
- ½ red onion
- ¼ tsp chili powder
- 2 tablespoons olive oil

## DIRECTIONS

1. In a bowl beat eggs with parsley, chili powder and salt
2. In a skillet heat olive oil and sauté onion for 2-3 minutes

3. Add egg mixture to the onions and cook for 4-5 minutes

4. When ready remove from heat and serve

# BREAKFAST ENCHILADAS

Serves:        **2**
Prep Time:   **10**   Minutes

Cook Time:   **20**   Minutes

Total Time:   **30**   Minutes

## INGREDIENTS

- 6 eggs
- ¼ cup coconut milk
- black pepper
- 2 tablespoons olive oil
- 4 slices bacon
- 1 cup baby spinach
- 1 cup black beans
- 1 cup tomatoes
- ¼ cup enchilada sauce
- ¼ cup cheddar cheese

## DIRECTIONS

1. In a bowl beat eggs with salt and set aside

2. In a pan melt butter and pour ½ cup egg mixture

3. Cook for 3-4 minutes

4. In a skillet cook bacon until crispy, add black beans, spinach and tomatoes, cook for 4-5 minutes

5. Lay egg tortilla on a cutting board and fill with spinach mixture, bacon and roll

6. In a pan spread enchilada sauce, add enchiladas and bake until cheese is melted

7. Serve when ready

# STUFFED PEPPERS

Serves:        **2**
Prep Time:    **10**   Minutes

Cook Time:   **40**   Minutes

Total Time:   **50**   Minutes

## INGREDIENTS

- 2 bell peppers
- 6 eggs
- ¼ cup coconut milk
- 2 slices bacon
- 1 cup cheddar cheese
- 1 tablespoon chives

## DIRECTIONS

1. Place peppers in a baking dish and cut side up
2. In a bowl beat eggs and combine with the rest of the ingredients
3. Pour egg mixture into peppers
4. Bake at 400 F for 30-35 minutes

5. When ready remove from the oven and serve

# AMERICAN PANCAKES

Serves:          **4**

Prep Time:    **10**   Minutes

Cook Time:    **10**   Minutes

Total Time:    **20**   Minutes

## INGREDIENTS

- ¼ lb. plain flour
- 1 tsp baking powder
- ¼ tsp salt
- 1 tablespoon brown sugar
- 150 ml milk
- 1 egg
- 1 tablespoon olive oil

## DIRECTIONS

1. In a bowl combine salt, sugar and baking powder
2. In another bowl combine milk and egg
3. Pour the milk mixture over flour mixture and mix well

4. In a pan heat olive oil and pour ¼ mixture
5. Cook for 1-2 minutes per side
6. When ready remove from heat and serve

# BLUEBERRY PANCAKES

Serves:       **4**
Prep Time:    **10**   Minutes

Cook Time:    **10**   Minutes

Total Time:   **20**   Minutes

## INGREDIENTS

- 100 ml double cream
- 4 tablespoons almond butter
- ¼ cup blueberries
- 4 ready-made pancakes

## DIRECTIONS

1. **Whip the cream until peaks forms**
2. **Pour almond butter and blueberries over pancakes**
3. **Roll and serve**

# DUCK PANCAKES

Serves: **4**

Prep Time: **5** Minutes

Cook Time: **15** Minutes

Total Time: **20** Minutes

## INGREDIENTS

- 4 duck breasts
- ¼ tsp Chinese spice
- 1 tablespoon sesame oil
- 3 oz. hoisin sauce
- 4-6 ready-made pancakes
- 1 bunch onions
- ¼ cucumber

## DIRECTIONS

1. Cut the duck breasts into thin strips and toss with spices
2. In a frying pan heat sesame oil add hoisin sauce and fry the duck breast for 4-5 minutes
3. Transfer duck to a plate

4. Over pancakes add onion, cucumber and duck breast
5. Wrap pancakes and serve

Serves:        *4*

Prep Time:   *10*   Minutes

Cook Time:   *20*   Minutes

Total Time:  *30*   Minutes

## INGREDIENTS

- 4 oz. buttermilk
- 150m flour
- 1 tsp baking powder
- 2 eggs
- 1 tablespoon olive oil

## DIRECTIONS

1. In a bowl combine all ingredients together
2. In a pan heat olive oil and pour ¼ mixture
3. Cook for 1-2 minutes per side
4. When ready remove from heat and serve

| Serves: | **8-12** | |
|---|---|---|
| Prep Time: | **10** | Minutes |
| Cook Time: | **20** | Minutes |
| Total Time: | **30** | Minutes |

## INGREDIENTS

- 2 cups all-purpose flour
- 1 tsp baking powder
- ¼ tsp salt
- ¼ cup brown sugar
- ¼ cup soy milk
- ¼ cup applesauce
- 1 cup blueberries

## DIRECTIONS

1. In a bowl combine dry ingredients
2. In another bowl combine wet ingredients
3. Fold the wet mixture into the dry mixture and mix well

4. Add blueberries and pour mixture into 8-12 muffin cups

5. Bake at 375 F for 18-20 minutes or until golden brown

6. When ready remove from heat and serve

# BANANA MUFFINS

Serves: **8**

Prep Time: **10** Minutes

Cook Time: **30** Minutes

Total Time: **40** Minutes

## INGREDIENTS

- 2 cups all-purpose flour
- ¼ tsp baking soda
- ¼ cup brown sugar
- ¼ tsp cinnamon
- ¼ cup olive oil
- ¼ cup coconut milk
- 2 eggs
- ¼ tsp vanilla extract

## DIRECTIONS

1. In a bowl combine dry ingredients
2. In another bowl combine wet ingredients

3. Fold the wet mixture into the dry mixture and mix well

4. Pour mixture into 8-12 muffin cups

5. Bake at 400 F for 20-25 minutes or until golden brown

6. When ready remove from heat and serve

# CHOCOLATE MUFFINS

Serves: **8**

Prep Time: **10** Minutes

Cook Time: **30** Minutes

Total Time: **40** Minutes

## INGREDIENTS

- 1 cup mashed banana
- ¼ cup sugar
- ¼ cup butter
- 2 eggs
- ½ cup cocoa powder
- 1 tsp baking powder
- 1 cup chocolate chips

## DIRECTIONS

1. In a bowl combine dry ingredients
2. In another bowl combine wet ingredients
3. Fold the wet mixture into the dry mixture and mix well

4. Fold in chocolate chips and pour mixture into 8-12 muffin cups

5. Bake at 375 F for 20-25 minutes or until golden brown

6. When ready remove from heat and serve

# PUMPKIN MUFFINS

Serves: **4**

Prep Time: **10** Minutes

Cook Time: **30** Minutes

Total Time: **40** Minutes

## INGREDIENTS

- ¼ cup coconut flour
- 1 tsp baking powder
- ¼ tsp salt
- 1 tsp cinnamon
- 1 tsp ginger
- ¼ tsp nutmeg
- ¼ tsp cloves
- 1 cup pumpkin puree
- ¼ coconut sugar
- 4 eggs
- 1 tsp chocolate chips

## DIRECTIONS

1. In a bowl combine dry ingredients
2. In another bowl combine wet ingredients
3. Fold the wet mixture into the dry mixture and mix well
4. Fold in chocolate chips and pour mixture into 8-12 muffin cups
5. Bake at 400 F for 20-25 minutes or until golden brown
6. When ready remove from heat and serve

# CHERRY-ALMOND OATMEAL

Serves:          *1*
Prep Time:   *10*   Minutes

Cook Time:   *10*   Minutes

Total Time:   *20*   Minutes

## INGREDIENTS

- ¼ cup gluten free oats
- ¼ cup water
- ¼ cup almond milk
- 1 banana
- 1 tablespoon brown sugar
- ¼ tsp vanilla extract
- ½ cup cherries
- ¼ cup almonds

## DIRECTIONS

1. In a saucepan add oats, water, banana, milk and cook for 4-5 minutes
2. When ready remove from heat and add remaining ingredients

3. Mix well and serve

# BANANA OATMEAL

Serves:        **2**
Prep Time:    **5**   Minutes

Cook Time:   **10**  Minutes

Total Time:  **15**  Minutes

## INGREDIENTS

- 1 cup oats
- 2 cup almond milk
- 1 tablespoon maple syrup
- 1 banana
- 1 tsp vanilla extract
- ¼ tsp cinnamon
- 1 tablespoon chia seeds

## DIRECTIONS

1. Place all ingredients into a saucepan and bring to a boil
2. Simmer for 5-6 minutes
3. When ready remove from heat

4. Transfer to a bowl, top with walnuts and serve

# STRAWBERRIES OATMEAL

Serves:          2

Prep Time:     5    Minutes

Cook Time:    10   Minutes

Total Time:    15   Minutes

## INGREDIENTS

- 2 cups oats
- 1 cup strawberries
- 1 tablespoon chia seeds
- 1 banana
- 2 cups almond milk
- 1 tablespoon maple syrup

## DIRECTIONS

1. Mash banana and strawberries together, set aside
2. In a saucepan add the rest of the ingredients and bring to a boil
3. Reduce heat and cook for 4-5 minutes
4. When ready transfer to the mashed banana mixture and mix well

5. Serve when ready

*LUNCH*

## CAULIFLOWER STEAKS WITH LEMON SAUCE

Serves:         *4*
Prep Time:  *10*  Minutes

Cook Time:  *10*  Minutes

Total Time:  *20*  Minutes

### INGREDIENTS

- 1 head cauliflower
- 2 tablespoons olive oil
- 2 tsp paprika

### LEMON SAUCE
- 1 cup parsley leaves
- ¼ cup mint leaves
- 1 garlic clove
- ¼ cup olive oil
- ¼ cup green onion
- Juice of 1 lemon

## DIRECTIONS

1. In a blender add all ingredients for the lemon sauce and blend until smooth
2. For the cauliflower steak, cut cauliflower into thick slices and rub with olive oil
3. Sprinkle with spices and place the cauliflower in a skillet
4. Cook for 4-5 minutes per side
5. When ready remove and serve with lemon sauce

Serves:        **4**

Prep Time:   **10**  Minutes

Cook Time:   **30**  Minutes

Total Time:   **40**  Minutes

## INGREDIENTS

- 2 tablespoons olive oil
- salt
- 2 scallions
- ¼ cup cilantro
- 1 head cauliflower
- 1 tablespoon sesame seeds

## SAUCE

- 1 tablespoon rice wine vinegar
- 1 tablespoon ginger
- 1 tsp olive oil
- 1 tablespoon soy sauce
- 1 tablespoon hoisin sauce

## DIRECTIONS

1. In a bowl combine all sauce ingredients together and mix well

2. For the cauliflower heat the olive oil in a skillet and add the cauliflower

3. Add salt, sesame seeds and cook for 4-5 minutes

4. When ready remove from heat, add cilantro and stir to combine

5. Serve with sauce

# RICE, KALE AND AVOCADO BOWL

Serves:         *2*
Prep Time:   *10*  Minutes

Cook Time:  *20*  Minutes

Total Time:  *30*  Minutes

## INGREDIENTS

- 1 cup rice
- 1 garlic clove
- 1 tablespoon rice vinegar
- 2 cups vegetable broth
- pinch of salt
- pinch of pepper
- 2 tablespoons
- 1 bunch kale
- 1 bunch kale
- 1 avocado

## DIRECTIONS

1. In a pot stir in broth, rice and garlic

2. Bring to a simmer for and cook until liquid is evaporated

3. When ready toss rice with salt, pepper and vinegar

4. In another books toss kale with olive oil

5. Add kale and avocado slices to the rice

6. Serve when ready

# CHICKEN MEATBALLS AND CAULIFLOWER RICE

Serves:       **4**

Prep Time:    **10**  Minutes

Cook Time:    **30**  Minutes

Total Time:   **40**  Minutes

## INGREDIENTS

- ¼ cup red onion
- 1 lb. ground chicken
- 1 tablespoon mustard
- ¼ tsp black pepper
- 1 tablespoon olive oil
- 1 garlic clove
- ¼ cup parsley
- pinch of salt

## SAUCE

- 1 cup parsley
- 1 can coconut milk
- 2 scallions
- zest of 1 lemon

-   1 cup ready-made cauliflower rice

## DIRECTIONS

1.  In a skillet heat olive oil and sauté onion and garlic for 3-4 minutes
2.  Remove sautéed onion and garlic to a bowl
3.  Stir in parsley, mustard, chicken, seasoning and mix well
4.  Form balls from the mixture and place on a baking sheet
5.  Bake at 400 F for 20 minutes
6.  When ready remove from the oven and set aside
7.  In a blender add all ingredients for the sauce and blend
8.  Top the meatballs with sauce and cauliflower rice and serve

# PINEAPPLE CHICKEN AND LETTUCE WRAPS

Serves:      **2**

Prep Time:   **10**  Minutes

Cook Time:   **20**  Minutes

Total Time:  **30**  Minutes

## INGREDIENTS

- 2 cups cooked chicken
- 1 tablespoon olive oil
- ¼ tsp paprika
- 1 tablespoon lime juice
- ¼ tsp garlic powder
- ¼ tsp salt
- 1 cup pineapple cubes
- 8 lettuce wraps

## DIRECTIONS

1. In a bowl combine garlic powder, lime juice, paprika, olive oil and lime juice
2. In your lettuce wraps add pineapple cubes, chicken and top with lime mixture

3. Serve when ready

# ROASTED SALMON WITH POTATOES

Serves:         **4**

Prep Time:   **10**   Minutes

Cook Time:   **35**   Minutes

Total Time:   **45**   Minutes

## INGREDIENTS

- 1 lb. potatoes
- 1 tsp lemon juice
- 4 salmon fillets
- ¼ tsp paprika
- 2 tablespoons olive oil

## DIRECTIONS

1. Bake the potatoes at 375 F for 20-25 minutes
2. Rub the salmon fillets with paprika and olive oil
3. Bake the fish until golden brown
4. When ready from the oven and serve with baked potatoes and lemon juice

# GUT ENERGY BOOSTING BOWL

Serves:          **1**

Prep Time:    **5**    Minutes

Cook Time:    **5**    Minutes

Total Time:   **10**   Minutes

## INGREDIENTS

- 2 cups kale
- 1 tablespoon olive oil
- 1 avocado
- ¼ cup carrot
- ½ cup beans
- ¼ cup cabbage
- 1 cup baked potatoes

## DIRECTIONS

1. In a bowl add all ingredients together
2. Drizzle olive oil and salt and mix well
3. Serve when ready

Serves: **2**
Prep Time: **5** Minutes
Cook Time: **10** Minutes
Total Time: **15** Minutes

## INGREDIENTS

- 2 zucchinis
- pinch of salt
- 2 avocados
- 2 tablespoons olive oil
- 2 eggs
- 1 tablespoon olive oil

## DIRECTIONS

1. In a bowl toss the zucchini noodles with olive oil
2. Season and transfer to a baking sheet
3. Crack an egg over each portion
4. Bake for 8-10 minutes at 375 F

5.  When ready remove from the oven and serve
    with avocado slices

Serves: **4**

Prep Time: **10** Minutes

Cook Time: **30** Minutes

Total Time: **40** Minutes

## INGREDIENTS

- 1 tablespoon olive oil
- 1 tablespoon honey
- 2 red bell peppers
- 2 carrots
- ¼ cup parsley
- 1 lb. chicken breast
- 2 onions

## DIRECTIONS

1. Place the chicken onto a baking sheet
2. Add the rest of the ingredients to the chicken breast
3. Drizzle olive oil over chicken and veggies

4. Bake at 375 F for 25-30 minutes or until the vegetables are tender

5. When ready remove from the oven and serve

Serves: **2**

Prep Time: **10** Minutes

Cook Time: **20** Minutes

Total Time: **30** Minutes

## INGREDIENTS

- 1 tablespoon cornstarch
- 1 garlic clove
- ¼ cup olive oil
- ¼ head broccoli
- ¼ cup show peas
- ½ cup carrots
- ¼ cup green beans
- 1 tablespoon soy sauce
- ½ cup onion

## DIRECTIONS

1. In a bowl combine garlic, olive oil, cornstarch and mix well

2. Add the rest of the ingredients and toss to coat
3. In a skillet cook vegetables mixture until tender
4. When ready transfer to a plate garnish with ginger and serve

# WALDORF SALAD

Serves: **2**

Prep Time: **5** Minutes

Cook Time: **5** Minutes

Total Time: **10** Minutes

## INGREDIENTS

- 1 tablespoon mayonnaise
- 1 tablespoon lemon juice
- 1 apple
- 1 cup red grapes
- ½ cup cranberries
- ½ cup walnuts
- 12 cup celery
- 6 lettuce leaves

## DIRECTIONS

1. In a bowl mix all ingredients and mix well
2. Serve with dressing

# CRANBERRY SALAD

Serves:         **2**
Prep Time:   **5**   Minutes

Cook Time:   **5**   Minutes

Total Time:  **10**  Minutes

## INGREDIENTS

- 1 can unsweetened pineapple
- 1 package cherry gelatin
- 1 tablespoon lemon juice
- ½ cup artificial sweetener
- 1 cup cranberries
- 1 orange
- 1 cup celery
- ½ cup pecans

## DIRECTIONS

1. In a bowl mix all ingredients and mix well
2. Serve with dressing

Serves:         2
Prep Time:    5    Minutes

Cook Time:    5    Minutes

Total Time:   10   Minutes

## INGREDIENTS

- ¼ lb. asparagus
- 1 zucchini
- 1 yellow squash
- ¼ red onion
- 1 red bell pepper
- ¼ cup olive oil
- ¼ cup red wine vinegar
- 2 garlic cloves
- Salt

## DIRECTIONS

1. Cut into thin strips and grill all vegetables
2. In a bowl mix all ingredients and mix well

3. Serve with salad dressing

Serves:         2
Prep Time:   5   Minutes

Cook Time:   5   Minutes

Total Time:  10  Minutes

## INGREDIENTS

- 2 lb. cabbage
- 2 carrots
- 2 beets
- 2 garlic cloves
- ¼ tsp black pepper
- ¼ cup olive oil

## DIRECTIONS

1. In a bowl mix all ingredients and mix well
2. Serve with dressing

# ROQUEFORT SALAD

Serves: **2**
Prep Time: **5** Minutes

Cook Time: **5** Minutes

Total Time: **10** Minutes

## INGREDIENTS

- 1 head leaf lettuce
- 2 pears
- 4 oz. Roquefort cheese
- 1 avocado
- ¼ cup green onions
- ¼ cup pecans
- ¼ cup olive oil
- 1 tsp mustard
- 1 garlic clove
- ¼ tsp salt

## DIRECTIONS

1. In a bowl mix all ingredients and mix well

2. Serve with dressing

# BLACK BEAN SALAD

Serves:       2

Prep Time:    5    Minutes

Cook Time:    5    Minutes

Total Time:   *10*   Minutes

## INGREDIENTS

- 1 can black beans
- 1 can corn
- 4 green onion
- 1 red bell pepper
- 2 tomatoes
- 1 lime
- ¼ cup salad dressing

## DIRECTIONS

1. In a bowl mix all ingredients and mix well
2. Serve with dressing

# CRANBERRY SALAD

Serves:        **2**

Prep Time:     **5**   Minutes

Cook Time:     **5**   Minutes

Total Time:    **10**  Minutes

## INGREDIENTS

- 1 can unsweetened pineapple
- 1 package cherry gelatin
- 1 tablespoon lemon juice
- ½ cup artificial sweetener
- 1 cup cranberries
- 1 orange
- 1 cup celery
- ½ cup pecans

## DIRECTIONS

1. In a bowl mix all ingredients and mix well
2. Serve with dressing

Serves:      **2**

Prep Time:   **5**   Minutes

Cook Time:   **5**   Minutes

Total Time:   **10**   Minutes

## INGREDIENTS

- 2 cups white beans
- ¼ can artichoke hearts
- ¼ cup red bell pepper
- ¼ cup black olives
- ½ cup red onion
- ¼ cup parsley
- Mint leaves
- ¼ cup olive oil

## DIRECTIONS

1. In a bowl mix all ingredients and mix well
2. Serve with dressing

# SAUERKRAUT SALAD

Serves:        **2**

Prep Time:   **5**   Minutes

Cook Time:   **5**   Minutes

Total Time:  **10**  Minutes

## INGREDIENTS

- 1-quart sauerkraut
- ¼ onion
- 3 celery stalks
- 1 red bell pepper
- ½ carrot
- 1 tsp mustard
- ¼ cup apple cider vinegar
- Salt

## DIRECTIONS

1. In a bowl mix all ingredients and mix well
2. Serve with dressing

# JICAMA SLAW

Serves:         2
Prep Time:    5    Minutes
Cook Time:    5    Minutes
Total Time:  *10*   Minutes

## INGREDIENTS

- 1 green cabbage
- 1 carrot
- 1 cup jicama
- 1 tablespoon sesame seeds
- 1 tablespoon apple cider vinegar
- 1 tablespoon olive oil
- ½ cup mayonnaise

## DIRECTIONS

1. In a bowl mix all ingredients and mix well
2. Serve with dressing

## CHICKPEA PASTA WITH GREEN PEAS

Serves: **4**

Prep Time: **10** Minutes

Cook Time: **20** Minutes

Total Time: **30** Minutes

## INGREDIENTS

- 1 oz. chickpea spaghetti
- ½ cup green peas
- 1 tablespoon olive oil
- 1 garlic clove
- ½ tsp black pepper
- 1 tablespoon parsley
- 1 tsp lemon zest

## DIRECTIONS

1. Cook pasta until al dente
2. Add green peas and cook until tender

3. In a skillet heat olive oil, add garlic, pepper, salt and pasta mixture, cook for 2-3 minutes

4. Stir in lemon zest, parsley and mix

5. When ready remove from heat and serve

# ROASTED CHICKPEAS

Serves:         2

Prep Time:   **10**   Minutes

Cook Time:   **30**   Minutes

Total Time:   **40**   Minutes

## INGREDIENTS

- 1 can chickpeas
- 1 tablespoon olive oil
- ¼ tsp black pepper
- ¼ tsp salt

## DIRECTIONS

1. Spread chickpeas on a baking sheet
2. Drizzle olive oil, black pepper and salt
3. Bake at 425 F for 25-30 minutes
4. When ready remove from the oven and serve

SIMPLE BULGUR

Serves: **2**
Prep Time: **5** Minutes

Cook Time: **15** Minutes

Total Time: **20** Minutes

## INGREDIENTS

- 1 cup water
- ½ cup bulgur
- 1 tsp olive oil
- ¼ tsp salt

## DIRECTIONS

1. In a saucepan bring water to a boil
2. Stir in bulgur and simmer for 12-15 minutes
3. When ready remove from heat and sprinkle olive oil and salt
4. Serve when ready

# SLOW COOKER QUINOA CURRY

Serves:          **6**
Prep Time:    **10**   Minutes

Cook Time:    **4**    Hours

Total Time:   **4**    Hours 10 Minutes

## INGREDIENTS

- 1 sweet potato
- 1 broccoli
- ¼ red onion
- 12 oz. chickpeas
- 1 can tomatoes
- 400 ml coconut milk
- 1 tsp tamari sauce
- ¼ tsp chili flakes

## DIRECTIONS

1. Place all the ingredients in a slow cooker
2. Cook on low heat for 4 hours or until vegetables are tender

3. When ready remove from the slow cooker and serve

# ROASTED BROCCOLI

Serves:        **6**

Prep Time:    **10**   Minutes

Cook Time:   **20**   Minutes

Total Time:   **30**   Minutes

## INGREDIENTS

- 2 heads broccoli
- 2 tablespoons sesame oil
- 2 garlic cloves
- ¼ tsp black pepper
- ¼ tsp salt

## DIRECTIONS

1. In a bowl toss broccoli with sesame oil, garlic, salt and black pepper
2. Spread broccoli on a baking sheet
3. Bake at 375 F for 15-20 minutes or until broccoli is tender
4. When ready remove from the oven and serve

# SPICY SHRIMP

Serves:          **4**

Prep Time:   **10**   Minutes

Cook Time:   **30**   Minutes

Total Time:  **40**   Minutes

## INGREDIENTS

- 1 cup ready-made cauliflower rice
- 1 cup avocado
- 1 cup cooked shrimp
- 1 tablespoon cilantro
- 1 tablespoon coconut amions
- 1 tablespoon sriracha sauce
- ¼ tsp smoked paprika

## DIRECTIONS

1. In a bowl mash avocado, stir in cilantro, coconut aminos, smoked paprika and mix well
2. Serve avocado mixture with cauliflower rice, shrimp and shrimp

# EMERALD SOUP

Serves:          **4**

Prep Time:    **5**    Minutes

Cook Time:   **10**   Minutes

Total Time:   **15**   Minutes

## INGREDIENTS

- 1 cucumber
- ½ avocado
- ½ cilantro
- 1 bunch spinach
- Juice of 1 lemon
- ¼ cup coconut aminos
- 1 L water
- salt

## DIRECTIONS

1. Place all ingredients in a blender and blend until smooth
2. Refrigerate soup for 2-3 hours

3. Serve when ready

CHICKEN CURRY

Serves:        2
Prep Time:    5   Minutes

Cook Time:   20  Minutes

Total Time:   25  Minutes

## INGREDIENTS

- 1 tablespoon olive oil
- 1 clove garlic
- 1 potato
- ¼ cup green onion
- 2 celery stalks
- 1 chicken breast
- ¼ tablespoon turmeric
- ¼ tsp coriander
- ¼ tsp garlic powder

## DIRECTIONS

1. In a skillet heat olive oil and sauté garlic and green onion

2. Add coriander, turmeric and garlic powder and cook for 1-2 minutes

3. Add the rest of the ingredients and bring to a simmer

4. Cook until most of the liquid has evaporated

5. When ready remove and serve

# LENTIL SOUP

Serves: **4-6**

Prep Time: **10** Minutes

Cook Time: **30** Minutes

Total Time: **40** Minutes

## INGREDIENTS

- 1 tablespoon sesame oil
- ½ cup red onion
- ½ cup celery
- ¼ cup turnip
- 1 tsp salt
- 1 tsp black pepper
- 1 cup green lentils
- 1 cup red lentils
- 1 tsp cumin
- 2 cups vegetable broth
- 1 cup water
- 1 cup coconut milk
- 2 cups potato

## DIRECTIONS

1. In a stockpot sauté celery, potato, garlic, turnip for 4-5 minutes

2. Add black pepper, lentils, water, milk, broth, and bring to a simmer for 20 minutes

3. Add spices and remaining ingredients and cook for another 5-10 minutes

4. When ready remove from heat and serve

# PURPLE SOUP

Serves: **4**

Prep Time: **10** Minutes

Cook Time: **40** Minutes

Total Time: **50** Minutes

## INGREDIENTS

- ½ red onion
- 1 lb. purple sweet potato
- 2 cups vegetables broth
- ¼ tsp salt
- ½ cup almond milk
- ¼ carrot
- 1 tablespoon olive oil

## DIRECTIONS

1. In a pot heat olive oil and add sauté onion for 4-5 minutes
2. Add sweet potato to the pot and vegetable broth
3. Bring to a boil and simmer for 30-35 minutes, or until the liquid is partially evaporated

4. Add remaining ingredients, excepting almond milk, and cook until potatoes are soft

5. When ready blend soup and add almond milk

6. Add salt and serve

# SMOOTHIES

## PEANUT BUTTER & BANANA SMOOTHIE

Serves:        **1**

Prep Time:    **5**   Minutes

Cook Time:    **5**   Minutes

Total Time:   **10**   Minutes

### INGREDIENTS

- 1 banana
- 1 cup coconut milk
- ¼ cup peanut butter
- 1 tablespoon honey
- 1 cup ice

### DIRECTIONS

1. In a blender place all ingredients and blend until smooth

2.  Pour smoothie in a glass and serve

Serves:       *1*
Prep Time:    *5*   Minutes

Cook Time:    *5*   Minutes

Total Time:   *10*  Minutes

## INGREDIENTS

- 1 banana
- 1 cup grapes
- ¼ cup Greek yogurt
- ¼ apple
- 1 cup baby spinach

## DIRECTIONS

1. In a blender place all ingredients and blend until smooth
2. Pour smoothie in a glass and serve

# PINEAPPLE-CARROT SMOOTHIE

Serves:       *1*
Prep Time:   *5*   Minutes

Cook Time:   *5*   Minutes

Total Time:  *10*  Minutes

## INGREDIENTS

- 6 oz. water
- 1 cup pineapple
- 1 orange
- 1 carrot
- 1 tablespoon chia seeds
- ½ tsp ginger
- 1 handful baby spinach

## DIRECTIONS

1. In a blender place all ingredients and blend until smooth
2. Pour smoothie in a glass and serve

# KIWI-KALE SMOOTHIE

Serves:        **1**

Prep Time:    **5**   Minutes

Cook Time:    **5**   Minutes

Total Time:   **10**  Minutes

## INGREDIENTS

- 4 oz. water
- 1 mango
- 1 kiwifruit
- 1 cup kale

## DIRECTIONS

1. In a blender place all ingredients and blend until smooth
2. Pour smoothie in a glass and serve

Serves:        *1*

Prep Time:    *5*   Minutes

Cook Time:   *5*   Minutes

Total Time:   *10*   Minutes

## INGREDIENTS

- 1 cup ice
- 1 cup baby spinach
- 1 cup pineapple
- 1 banana
- ½ cup orange
- mint leaves
- ¼ lemon juice
- ¼ lime juice

## DIRECTIONS

1. In a blender place all ingredients and blend until smooth
2. Pour smoothie in a glass and serve

# OATMEAL BREAKFAST SMOOTHIE

Serves:        *1*

Prep Time:   *5*   Minutes

Cook Time:   *5*   Minutes

Total Time:   *10*   Minutes

## INGREDIENTS

- 1 cup soy milk
- ¼ cup oats
- 1 banana
- 1 cup strawberries
- ¼ tsp vanilla extract
- 1 tsp cinnamon

## DIRECTIONS

1. In a blender place all ingredients and blend until smooth
2. Pour smoothie in a glass and serve

# MATCHA SMOOTHIE

Serves:        *1*

Prep Time:    *5*   Minutes

Cook Time:   *5*   Minutes

Total Time:   *10*   Minutes

## INGREDIENTS

- 1 cup mango
- ¼ cup kale
- 2 tablespoons black beans
- 1 tablespoon coconut flakes
- ¼ tsp matcha powder
- 1 cup ice

## DIRECTIONS

1. In a blender place all ingredients and blend until smooth
2. Pour smoothie in a glass and serve

# CALIFORNIA SMOOTHIE

Serves: **1**

Prep Time: **5** Minutes

Cook Time: **5** Minutes

Total Time: **10** Minutes

## INGREDIENTS

- 1 cup strawberries
- 1 cup lemon yogurt
- ¼ cup lime juice
- ½ cup orange juice

## DIRECTIONS

1. In a blender place all ingredients and blend until smooth
2. Pour smoothie in a glass and serve

Serves:      **1**

Prep Time:   **5**   Minutes

Cook Time:   **5**   Minutes

Total Time:  **10**  Minutes

INGREDIENTS

- 1 cup pineapple
- Ginger
- ¼ cup coconut milk
- 1 tablespoon brown sugar
- ¼ cup orange juice

**DIRECTIONS**

1. In a blender place all ingredients and blend until smooth
2. Pour smoothie in a glass and serve

# GRAPEFRUIT SMOOTHIE

Serves:      **1**

Prep Time:   **5**   Minutes

Cook Time:   **5**   Minutes

Total Time:  **10**  Minutes

## INGREDIENTS

- 2 grapefruits
- 1 cup ice
- 2 oz spinach
- ¼ inch ginger root
- 1 tsp flax seeds

## DIRECTIONS

1. In a blender place all ingredients and blend until smooth
2. Pour smoothie in a glass and serve

**THANK YOU FOR READING THIS BOOK!**

Made in the USA
Middletown, DE
11 February 2023

24614699R00061